LIZ EARLE'S
QUICK GUIDES

Detox

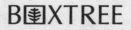

B⬆XTREE

Advice to the Reader
Before following any dietary advice contained in this book, it is
recommended that you consult your doctor if you suffer from any health
problems or special condition or are in any doubt.

First published in Great Britain in 1995 by Boxtree Limited,
Broadwall House, 21 Broadwall, London SE1 9PL

The right of Liz Earle to be identified as Author of this Work has
been asserted by her in accordance with the Copyright, Designs and
Patents Act 1988

10 9 8 7 6 5 4 3 2 1

ISBN: 1 85283 979 1

Text design by Blackjacks
Cover design by Hammond Hammond

Printed and Bound in Great Britain by Cox & Wyman Ltd.,
Reading, Berkshire

A CIP catalogue entry for this book is available from
the British Library

Contents

Acknowledgements 4

Introduction 5

1. Why We Need to Detox 7

2. How to Detox 17

3. Starting the Detox 31

4. The Detox Diet 35

5. Meal Plans 41

6. Detox Diet Boosters 51

7. Herbs and Supplements 61

8. Lymphatic Drainage 67

9. Aromatherapy Detox Massage 71

10. Exercise and Breathing 81

Glossary 89

Useful Addresses 91

Index 93

ACKNOWLEDGEMENTS

I am grateful to Sarah Hamilton-Fleming for helping to produce this book, and for the excellent advice from Maurice Hanssen. I am also indebted to the talented team at Boxtree and Claire Bowles Publicity for their unfailing enthusiasm and support.

Introduction

When I was first told that fasting on a fruit-only diet would give me more energy, or that giving up some of my favourite foods and cups of coffee would leave my skin glowing, I was sceptical. But the principles of detoxification are based on traditional 'cures' practised by European naturopaths for centuries. Giving up certain foods, or existing on fruit alone for twenty-four hours, is not hard, especially when the benefits are so great. I now give my system a regular detox boost – even if it is only over a weekend. It is the perfect way to revitalise the body, renew energy levels and restore glowing skin. A brief period of detox is also the perfect way to kick-start a healthy eating regime or a few months of intensive weight-loss. Whatever your reasons for choosing a detox programme, this *Quick Guide* gives you all you need to know about getting the best out of your body.

Liz Earle

1

Why We Need to Detox

Toxic substances invade our bodies every day, although most of us are unaware of the fact. 'All substances are poisons,' said Paracelsus, the Swiss father of toxicology, in the fifteenth century, and this is particularly true in our modern Western world. Most people know that cigarettes and heavy alcohol consumption are toxic, but few realise that much of the food which we consider to be good for us also contains toxins.

The majority of supermarket food is processed, and so is damaged in some way, to preserve it. Many foods are either smoked, salted, dried, pickled, chilled, refined, canned or chemically treated and all these processes alter the natural food in some way and often deplete it of many of its essential nutrients. When food is canned, vitamin C and many of the B vitamins are lost, while the sodium and potassium balance is often destroyed by added salt. The packaging itself can also be damaging. The aluminium in some cans can seep into the food while the cans are heated and sealed.

Many food additives are also toxic, some more than others, and some experts claim that additives such as aspartame, which is used as a sugar substitute, may be particularly harmful. According to naturopath Leon Chaitow, 'when aspartame is digested, it breaks down into methanol, better known as wood alcohol. After your enzymes have digested this, it may end up in your bloodstream as formaldehyde, a chemical which is used to preserve dead bodies, with unpredictable toxic effects.' However, it is reliably estimated that the first signs of a toxic effect from methanol are caused by consuming between 200 and 500mg of methanol per kilo of body weight. The manufacturer assures us that even those people who have large amounts of aspartame in their diet, such as diabetics, never consume anywhere near this amount. In fact, you would have to drink more than 600 cans of soft drink containing aspartame simultaneously to produce any toxic quantity of methanol. It is, nonetheless, a good idea to limit the amount of artificial additives, including aspartame, in your diet and these should be avoided altogether while on the detox diet.

Our bodies are probably most toxic after a time of indulgence, such as at Christmas, when most of us eat and drink large amounts of unhealthy food and alcohol. One of our New Year resolutions should always be to detoxify the body and get it back into good shape. Detoxing should only take a few days if it is done properly, and then we will be ready to start the New Year with a clear mind and body. We all go on the odd binge and this won't cause permanent damage to the system provided we make an effort to compensate for these lapses through a healthy detoxing diet. Even those who eat healthily and take regular exercise will need to give their body a spring clean every once in a while. However, detoxing is not simply a matter of eating more fruit and vegetables while maintaining all our bad habits, although it will help!

Unfortunately though, even fruit and vegetables are not free of artificial toxins, unless they are organically grown. Modern farming uses pesticides, insecticides, fungicides and herbicides to kill the insects, rodents and weeds which interfere with crop production. These pesticides are so powerful that they remain in the food, the soil and the water and, ultimately, in us. The production of meat, poultry and milk is equally unpleasant and unnatural. Poultry are continuously pumped with antibiotics to make them more resistant to disease. Many other farm animals are also given antibiotics and hormones to increase rapid growth. One result of this is that cows' milk may contain drug residues and contaminants as well as food-poisoning bacteria which can sometimes survive pasteurisation. There were many outbreaks of listeriosis (30 percent of cases are fatal) in pasteurised cheese in Britain in 1989.

When we look at the fresh vegetables and the smartly packaged foods in the supermarket, few of us are really aware of what has gone on behind the scenes to produce these products, and what the damaging effects of these processes are. Here are some important things to look for when buying food:

* Choose from the many organic fruit, vegetables, meat and dairy products available now – these are grown without the aid of pesticides and other toxic chemicals.

* Don't buy fruit and vegetables which are on display near a busy road as these will have been exposed to heavy-metal pollution from car exhaust fumes.

* Scrub all hard-skinned produce, such as apples and nectarines, in well-diluted washing-up liquid and then rinse well.

* Remove the outer leaves of leafy vegetables.

* Supplement your diet regularly with friendly bacteria such as acidophilus which is present in live yoghurt. This will reduce your chances of succumbing to attack from bugs such as salmonella and listeria.

It is not just food which is a source of toxins. Living in the modern Western world our bodies are continuously open to toxins through the air which we breathe. The atmosphere is full of pollutants from cars, from industrial chemicals and even many household appliances, which are highly carcinogenic.

These include petrochemical vapours, asbestos, pesticides, radon, sulphur and nitrogen dioxide.

We are all exposed to heavy-metal toxicity no matter what measures we take to avoid it. Exhaust fumes are the main source of lead but cigarette smoke is another key source. There is an increasing amount of evidence which suggests that high levels of lead in the body diminish our powers of concentration, lower our IQ, will increase the chance of miscarriage and birth defects and will generally speed up the ageing process. We are also exposed to heavy-metal toxicity in the form of mercury through our diet and dental fillings. Fungicides which are used to protect grains contain mercury and much of the fish that we eat comes from mercury-saturated seas. Mercury poisoning is very serious and its symptoms are blurred vision, headaches, dizziness and depression – even some brain tumours can also be caused by mercury poisoning. Another heavy metal which pervades our world is aluminium in the form of aluminium foil, aluminised salts, baking powder, toothpaste, cigarette filters, processed cheese, hot-water heaters, cosmetics and pharmaceuticals. Symptoms of aluminium poisoning include persistent indigestion and stomach upsets. Food cooked in aluminium saucepans absorbs aluminium which, when eaten, produces a gas in your stomach. This gas upsets the delicate pH of your whole digestive system which overburdens all your organs of detoxification. Smokers are continuously exposing themselves to another kind of heavy-metal toxin, cadmium. They have much higher levels of this metal in their livers than non-smokers. Traces of cadmium may also be found in tin cans, instant coffee, cola drinks, refined cereals and many processed meats. Cadmium poisoning can cause hypertension, brain haemorrhage and kidney and liver damage. A diet free of processed foods with a reasonable amount of vitamin D in the form of sunshine will help to counteract the ill-effects of too much cadmium in the system.

We also experience radiation from the sun, as well as from rural and urban landscapes in the form of granite and some building materials such as concrete, bricks and tiles. A small amount of radiation is not harmful to us, but in higher doses it can cause cancer. Sunlight, although essential for our health, is also very damaging in large doses and can cause skin cancer, as well as creating free-radicals inside us which in turn cause cell damage. Our best protection from the harmful rays of the sun is the ozone layer, but unfortunately this is diminishing because of the damaging pollutants that are continuously let loose into the atmosphere.

Here are some things that we can all do to limit the amount of pollution we create and how it affects us:

* Limit the amount you use your car either by walking, using public transport or sharing a vehicle.

* Fit your car with a catalytic converter so that you can use lead-free petrol.

* Use ozone-friendly aerosol sprays.

* Recycle packaging, separating glass, aluminium foil and plastic – some councils run a special recycling collection service.

* Always breathe through your nose instead of your mouth when in heavily polluted areas. The nose can filter some of the pollution so that it is not fully inhaled.

* Try to avoid industrial urban areas where there is a lot of traffic, especially in hot weather when the concentration of ground-level ozone is highest.

* Do not cook food in aluminium saucepans as the aluminium is absorbed by some foods. Use iron, stainless steel, enamel-lined, china, glass or earthenware saucepans instead.

* Protect yourself from the sun with high-protection sun creams or sit in the shade.

* Limit the amount of mucus-forming dairy and wheat products you eat as these increase lead absorption. Eat plenty of calcium in the form of millet, alfalfa, sesame seeds and parsley to help mop up any excess lead in the body.

* Drink plenty of mineral water and eat foods containing the antioxidant ACE vitamins: beta-carotene, vitamin C and vitamin E.

Our Modern Diet

Recent research has revealed that the health of a nation depends upon what people eat. For example Mediterranean people have a much lower risk of suffering from heart attacks and strokes than Britons, and this has been linked to a diet traditionally containing mostly fresh produce, lots of fish and olive oil which are high in essential fatty acids and other nutrients. The medical link between diet and health is now well established, but the food industry continuously produces highly processed, unhealthy products, often with evasive or misleading marketing. As a nation we may have a longer life expectancy than ever before, but serious diseases such as cardiovascular degeneration and high blood pressure, arthritis and cancer are occurring in humans earlier than ever. Many of these diseases in children have been linked to a deficient diet.

Allergy is one of the most common results of a bad diet and allergic reactions coupled with toxicity can be a deadly combination. Toxins in the body have to be dealt with by the immune system and the organs of detoxification: the liver, kidneys and skin. If you already have an allergy, these organs will be put under greater strain and with increased exposure to toxicity, your whole body may become sensitised and produce increasingly violent allergic reactions. The most common food allergies are caused by wheat, eggs and dairy produce. If you do have an allergic reaction to something you are eating, then try cutting out a particular type of food, such as dairy produce, from your diet to establish if that is the true cause.

Toxicity in the Office

Many modern offices, no matter how clean and plush they are, have a toxic atmosphere which is utterly undetectable. The United States Environmental Protection Agency claims that the air in some offices is a hundred times more polluted than the air outside. Air-conditioning and heating systems, which are supposed to be a source of comfort, are in fact a breeding ground for undesirable, sometimes lethal, fungi and bacteria, especially if they are regularly turned off at night and at weekends. Most of the toxicity in offices comes from the copying machine chemicals, carbon paper, paint and cleaning solvents, most of which release vapours of formaldehyde which is capable of causing skin rashes, nausea and menstrual irregularities. If you are frequently having headaches at work then a toxic atmosphere may be the cause. Instead of taking painkillers, take regular breaks from the office, if only for a minute or so each time, and drink plenty of mineral water.

Toxicity at Home

Even your home is not a safe haven from toxic substances, sometimes from seemingly innocent sources. The actual building you live in probably contains timber and damp-proofing treatments, paints, chipboards and plastic tiles, which are all a source of toxicity. Although there is little you can do to change this, you can at least watch for any allergic reactions that may occur when using household products, here are the toxic effects of some household objects:

* Paper kitchen towels contain formaldehyde to strengthen the paper, this can cause skin rashes, nausea and menstrual irregularities.

* Liquid detergents for washing dishes and clothes may contain calcium sodium edetate or phosphate compounds which can penetrate the skin and are toxic irritants.

* Many air fresheners contain carbolic acid and formaldehyde, as well as CFCs which damage the ozone layer.

* A germ killer in toilet cleaners called cresol can be easily absorbed through the skin and can damage major organs.

* The main ingredient of most cleaners is lye which is one of the most toxic substances known to man.

* The sodium phosphate or turpentine in furniture polish may penetrate the skin or be inhaled as vapour.

* Commercial floor cleaners containing the chemical lauryl dimethyl benzyl (ammonium chloride) may cause asthma.

Toxic Toiletries

Objects which we use every day to keep us feeling clean and fresh may also be toxic. Antiperspirants generally contain aluminium chlorohydrate which blocks the pores of the skin, preventing the body eliminating waste through the skin. Bicarbonate of soda can be used to keep the underarms dry instead. Simply rub a teaspoonful under the arms. Regular washing combined with the use of sweet-smelling essential oils can be used as an alternative to deodorants. Put a few drops of an essential oil you like into a small bottle of base oil such as avocado or grapeseed oil and massage into your armpits, when this is fully rubbed in, pat on a little bicarbonate of soda to keep them dry.

Even the stuff most of us brush our teeth with every day contains toxic substances such as ammonia, ethanol, formaldehyde and saccharine. A much better alternative is the bicarbonate of soda toothpastes which can now be bought.

There is a wealth of natural cosmetic and toiletry products available now and these are generally less toxic than those which are chemically formulated. If you have the time, you can make your own creams and ointments from essential oils and herbs. Instead of using an anti-dandruff shampoo, which treats your scalp with toxic chemicals, here is my recipe for a natural anti-dandruff hair tonic.

Anti-dandruff Hair Tonic

Make a strong nettle tea using 4 dessertspoons (40ml) of dried nettle leaves or 4 nettle herb tea bags. While the nettle tea is infusing, make a birch infusion by stirring 15ml (1 tablespoon) of fresh or dried birch leaves into a cupful of almost boiling water. Leave to steep for 30 minutes. When the two infusions are ready, mix together and pour into bottles. Apply to the hair and scalp two or three times a week, or use as a final hair rinse after washing (do not rinse out).

—— 2 ——

How to Detox

The Body's Fight Against Toxins

The body does not just passively absorb toxins, it makes a concerted effort to eliminate them, even while we are sleeping. The speed at which our body can deal with toxins depends on our age and general state of health. The younger and healthier you are, the more efficient your body will be at ridding itself of these unwanted substances, incurring less damage to your body. The complex process of detoxification involves the immune system (especially the white blood cells), the lungs, kidneys, liver, bowels and the skin. One of the main sources of toxic waste in your body are the bits of food which the body is unable to break down and convert into energy. Your body also creates its own waste when its cells die. Some parts of the cell such as amino acids and essential fatty acids are recycled by the liver and various enzymes, and can then be re-used. Any leftover waste is eliminated in urine and faeces, through exhalation or through perspiration via the skin.

The immune system copes with any irritant substances present in food or in the environment. For example if you are in a smoke-filled room, you are being damaged by free-radicals. To fight this attack, your immune system automatically responds by making your eyes water with a soothing antioxidant substance which neutralises the irritant toxins. Other toxins such as alcohol are not as easy to deal with and the body has to employ other organs such as the liver to make sure that they do not harm the body. However, regular consumption of large amounts of alcohol or other toxic substances can cause toxic overload, where the organ which attempts to eliminate the toxin is overwhelmed. The bowel is a key organ in the process of detoxifying your body. If its activity is blocked in some way by poor dietary habits causing constipation, then decaying food debris may become toxic and enter the bloodstream, slowly poisoning you. To deal with these loose toxins, another organ of elimination, such as the skin, will attempt to rid the body of them.

Homeostasis

The human body is like a wonderful self-generating machine. It heals and regulates itself through a process known as homeostasis. One of the key functions of homeostasis is to detoxify your body. The efficiency of these functions depends upon what you inherited through the genes of your parents and how you treat your body. Some people seem to cause endless abuse to their body and yet come out unscathed, while others are unable to cope with small amounts of toxins and stress. This factor is probably genetic. However, it is possible to improve your levels of homeostasis.

THE IMMUNE SYSTEM
The immune system is present everywhere in your body and there are many ways in which its function can be improved. The trace mineral selenium boosts its primary response by re-enforcing the body's natural enzyme defence mechanism. Extra vitamin C boosts its overall resistance to attack, and excess essential fatty acids can boost T- and B-cell function (these white blood cells – lymphocytes – together are responsible for creating antibodies and cell immunity). Forty-eight-hour water-only fasts can also boost immunity and have been shown to raise white blood cell counts.

THE LIVER

This important detoxifying organ has over 1,500 different functions from secreting bile to the formation of blood. It processes all foods (except for some fats) which have been absorbed by the intestines, before releasing them into the bloodstream. The liver also filters the blood, removing, deactivating or reprocessing toxins, wastes and bacteria, but if it is bombarded with too many toxins, its ability to detoxify will be diminished. However, the liver has a marvellous capacity to regenerate itself so even if you have consumed large amounts of alcohol and other toxins over the years, now is your chance to give it a fresh start with this detox programme. One of the best liver cleansers is dandelion; a coffee made from dandelion root and dandelion tea can both be obtained from health food shops.

THE LUNGS

Any toxic debris left in your internal system can be exhaled through the lungs. In fact, far more is passed this way than through urine. Toxic pollutants which are inhaled reach the bloodstream more quickly than those arriving via the digestive system in food as there is less filtering performed by the lungs. Your lungs are constantly flushing out carbon dioxide and carbonic acid wastes every time you breathe out. The way in which we breathe is actually very important although most of us pay little attention to this vital act. Always breathe through your nose, which filters some of the toxins, and exhale through your mouth, which is the best method of ridding your lungs of toxins.

Carbon monoxide in car exhaust fumes and nicotine from cigarette smoke are two of the biggest causes of cancer and cardiovascular disease in the Western world. These horrifying statistics could be changed by a general switch to a healthier lifestyle and by improving the body's ability to rid itself of toxins.

Your diet also affects your lungs. Some dietary therapists believe that dairy products, eggs, meat, refined foods and the gluten in wheat can all clog up the lungs. One of the best expectorants to clear the lungs is garlic, preferably fresh, although you can buy garlic capsules in health food shops. See the section on herbs on page 62 to discover which other herbs help to clear the lungs.

THE KIDNEYS

The action of the kidneys is twofold. They eliminate toxins from the blood through urine and they also salvage and re-absorb valuable nutrients which can be recycled for future use by the body. Our bodies are mainly filled with water and we eliminate about four and a half litres of water every day through the skin, the kidneys and the organs of elimination. Unfortunately, the efficiency of this filter effect diminishes with age or excessive toxicity due to diet, drugs or a toxic environment. Any weakening of the kidneys affects the heart, and may be a contributing factor in coronary heart disease. It is important never to ignore a full bladder as this will press down on the pelvic organs. Toxins can be flushed out by drinking large amounts of purified water and fruit and vegetable juices. Asparagus juice is a particularly good kidney cleanser, although pure water works well too.

THE SKIN

The skin acts as a marvellous back-up for the other organs of elimination. If these other organs are blocked or damaged in some way, then the skin comes to the rescue. If blemishes, pimples, boils or rashes appear on the face, this is a sign that your body is trying to rid itself of toxins. Instead of suppressing skin disorders, they should be allowed to 'come out' and looked upon as a sign that the body's internal biochemistry is in disarray. In the skin there are hundreds of thousands of sweat glands which act like mini kidneys, by detoxifying organs and cleansing the blood. In order for the skin to do its job properly, its pores need to be completely unblocked and that is why we should not wear deodorants and antiperspirants. One of the best ways to exfoliate the skin is by skin brushing (see page 67) or by an Epsom salt rub. The latter treatment should not be used if you have high blood pressure or a heart condition. Massage yourself all over with equal quantities of Epsom salts and almond oil with circular movements, working towards the heart. This should be repeated every couple of days before taking a bath with a tablespoonful of Epsom salts to help remove all dead skin cells or fungi, which may be blocking the pores of the skin. Epsom salts can be bought from good chemists.

THE INTESTINES AND MICRO-ORGANISMS
The food we eat passes from the stomach into the intestines where its nutrients are absorbed and the residue is left for elimination. There are literally hundreds of short-lived micro-organisms involved in this process. Living inside your intestines are about 400 different species of micro-organisms, some of which are wanted and some of which are harmful, and between them they weigh 35 pounds. Some of the good ones are friendly *Bifido-bacteria* and *Lactobacillus acidophilus* (this is also found in live yoghurt) which are brilliant agents of detoxification. They may help you to digest your food as well as stimulating peristaltic action (the movement which pushes the bowel contents along). They also control some of the unwanted bowel contents such as *Candida albicans*, a fungus which is primarily responsible for candidiasis (a yeast-like infection of the mouth, lungs, intestines, vagina, skin and nails).

THE BOWEL
The bowel shifts large amounts of waste daily but it can easily get clogged up through poor diet. If you think one bowel

movement a day is good then think again! Four-fifths of the food which you eat should be eliminated via the bowels and one bowel movement is probably not going to do the job. Constipation is not merely uncomfortable, it can be one of the sources of heart disease through the blood being poisoned by trapped waste, which in turn raises the level of cholesterol in the blood. Some of the food in our diet gets left behind in the colon causing a build-up of waste. Highly refined starches such as cakes, dairy produce, eggs, sugar and prescription drugs, together with a lack of fluid and fibre, are the main culprits.

LYMPHATICS

Lymph is a fluid derived from the blood and it is carried around the body via a vast network of vessels. The lymphatic drainage system interacts with the bloodstream through special ducts, and it depends mainly on the pump action of breathing, and the action of our muscles as they contract during use. Lymph passes through a series of filters (lymph nodes) before leaving a vital organ. Lymph vessels contain a huge amount of white blood cells which attack invaders and clean out waste. These key immune function agents are called lymphocytes and macrophages and they protect us against infection, cancer and toxicity. The B lymphocytes produce antibodies which attack any invaders while the T-cells actively hunt for foreign invading cells, bacteria, viruses and allergens. You can spot lymph nodes in your neck because they swell up when you have a cold or throat infection. They are also located in the armpits, groin and backs of the knees. The lymphatic drainage system plays an important part in the removal of waste, but it can become easily clogged by a diet which is too rich in red meat, dairy products, sugar, fried food and synthetic substances that the body finds difficult to deal with.

Signs of Toxicity

Your body will probably let you know when it is in need of a detox. Here are some of the symptoms you may be experiencing due to exposure to toxic substances:

* general tiredness and lack of energy

* headaches

* muscle aches

* digestive problems such as bloating, cramps, nausea and diarrhoea

* frequent infections in the upper respiratory tract (lungs etc) such as colds and 'flu

* poor skin condition

* cellulite

There are more obvious and severe symptoms of toxic overload, such as diarrhoea as a result of food poisoning and severe burning as a result of contact with bleach or other toxic household substances. Heavy-metal pollution in the air and water is fairly common, and you will certainly know when you are victim of this as it can produce headaches, hyperactivity, memory lapses and behavioural changes. It is important to treat the cause itself and not just the symptom. A painkiller may relieve the suffering of a headache but it is not doing your body any good. If you can find out what is causing the headaches, then you may be able to stop yourself from getting them in the first place.

Unless you lead a superbly healthy lifestyle, then you probably need to detoxify your body, regardless of whether you feel fine or not. We all expose our bodies to some toxins no matter how hard we try not to. Many people smoke cigarettes daily and yet feel fine, but this does not mean that the nicotine, cadmium, formaldehyde, carbon monoxide, sulphur dioxide and tar (to name but a few of their toxins) are not doing them any harm. If you are a smoker, think back to when you had your first cigarette. Your body probably reacted by making you cough and choke. When you repeat this toxic experience, the body adapts to it and reacts less violently as it becomes 'sensitised' to the substance. Eventually it learns to live with this regular dose of toxins through the supreme effort of your organs of detoxification. If you continue to smoke for a long time, the body becomes addicted to the nicotine, the ability to detoxify diminishes, and the result is disease or early death.

If you do have a life-threatening habit such as smoking or drinking large amounts of alcohol, you should make an effort to cut down on these substances and detoxify your body regularly, whether your body shows any signs of toxic overload or not. You will be amazed at how much better you feel afterwards.

Do You Have Toxic Overload?

Here is a quick quiz to establish the extent of the toxins in your body and which detox diet in this *Quick Guide* is best suited to you.

DIET

Give yourself 3 points if the answer to the question is true for you Regularly (twice weekly or more), 2 points if it is true for you Occasionally (once a week or less), and 1 point if it is Rarely true (once every few months).

1. Do you just have a cup of tea or coffee for breakfast instead of something more substantial?

2. Do you snack between meals on crisps, chocolate bars, biscuits and cakes?

3. Do you eat readily prepared meals from supermarkets that merely require reheating?

4. Do you drink canned drinks?

5. Do you eat tinned vegetables?

6. Do you eat fast food such as burgers and pizzas from restaurants?

7. Do you add salt to your food?

8. Do you not eat fresh fruit and vegetables every day?

9. Do you eat foods fried in butter or animal fats?

10. Do you re-use fat or cooking oil?

11. Do you eat full-fat dairy products such as cheese, milk and yoghurt?

12. Do you eat red meat?

13. Do you eat processed meat and fish products such as smoked ham or fish?

14. Do you eat more than two teaspoons of sugar, honey or syrup a day?

15. *Do you eat ice-cream?*

16. *Do you use sauces such as tomato ketchup and brown sauce?*

17. *Do you eat canned or dried fruit (which contains sulphur dioxide)?*

18. *Do you eat white bread, pasta and rice instead of the natural 'brown' varieties?*

19. *Do you eat processed cereals instead of sugarless muesli, granola or oatmeal?*

TOXIC STIMULANTS

Give yourself 3 points if your answer is Yes and 0 points if your answer is No.

1. *Do you drink more than one and a half glasses of wine, one pint of beer, or a measure of spirit daily?*

2. *Do you drink more than one cup of tea daily?*

3. *Do you drink more than one cup of coffee (even decaffeinated) daily?*

4. *Do you drink tap water?*

5. *Do you eat mostly non-organically grown fruit and vegetables?*

6. *Do you eat chocolate?*

7. *Do you eat mostly non-free-range meat, poultry and eggs?*

8. Does any of the food you eat contain added colourings or preservatives?

9. Do you smoke tobacco every day?

10. Do you smoke twenty or more cigarettes or five or more cigars a day?

11. Do you take any prescription drugs on a regular basis?

12. Do you take painkillers or other similar drugs on a regular basis?

ENVIRONMENT

Give yourself 3 points if your answer is Yes and 0 points if your answer is No.

1. Do you come in close contact with toxic chemicals at work?

2. Is your home or place of work air-conditioned, centrally heated or double glazed?

3. Do you work near to electrical machines such as computers?

4. Do you have synthetic or vinyl-backed furniture at home?

5. Do you use household cleaners and polishes daily?

6. Do you use chemical pesticides or fertiliser in your garden?

7. Do you swim in chlorinated water more than once a week?

8. Do you exercise on city roads more than twice a week?

9. *Do you live or work near a busy, main road or heavy industrial buildings such as power stations?*

Now it is time to add up your points and, depending on the total, find out just how toxic you are:

19–34 You have a very healthy diet and lifestyle and your body is probably able to cope with the small amount of toxins it is exposed to. However, as you are still exposed to some toxins, it is advisable that you boost your body's own detoxification processes with a good daily dose of the antioxidant ACE vitamins, A, C, and E.

35–75 You generally have a healthy diet consisting of lots of fresh fruit and vegetables, but you may sometimes enjoy processed food, unhealthy snacks and fast food. You probably do not give your body high doses of toxins through smoking or excessive drinking of alcohol, but you perhaps live or work in a fairly toxic environment. Those who scored between 60 and 75 have less healthy eating and lifestyle habits. To rid your body of any build-up of toxins and to boost your general health, you should follow the seven-day detox diet outlined in this *Quick Guide* (see page 35).

76–120 Your body is either in toxic overload or close to it! You may feel fine, but this is merely because your body's organs of detoxification have been working overtime to keep you that way and, sooner or later, these organs will not be able to cope with the steady flow of toxins. Your diet is poor, probably full of processed foods, red meat, full-fat dairy products, biscuits and crisps. You are also likely to smoke or drink too much, rely too heavily on drugs such as painkillers, and/or live or work in a heavily polluted area. The twenty-one-day detox diet (see page 38) is needed to rid your body of this steady build-up of toxins. However, this is only the start as you need to break your bad habits and develop a new healthier diet and lifestyle in the long term.

3

Starting the Detox

The process of detoxification is by no means easy and it involves a great deal of will power. To do it properly, you must begin with a two-day diet of only fruit and water and continue with a mainly raw food diet for the remainder of the time. You will also have to give up all stimulants such as tea, coffee and alcohol for that period, before embarking on a generally healthier diet in the long term. This should be combined with detoxification boosters such as skin brushing and aromatherapy massage. This clearly is no easy task for most of us who have unhealthy habits which are difficult to give up for any length of time. This is not like most weight-loss diets, where you can have the odd unhealthy snack or cup of coffee, the process of detoxification will only work properly if the diet is stuck to rigidly. The best thing about a detox diet is that it only lasts for a short time. But when you have finished, you will feel far fitter and healthier and will probably not wish to return to your toxic habits.

The time which you set aside for your detox is all important as it will contribute greatly to its success. Detoxing not only involves a great deal of will power, it depletes you of energy and may have other uncomfortable side-effects such as caffeine-withdrawal headaches. What with choosing your food carefully, skin brushing and massage, it involves a lot of time focused solely on you. This is difficult to accomplish if you have a demanding partner or family. You will find it difficult to live on fruit and water alone if you are having to cook meals for your family or if you have young children who sap your energy. The detox diet is equally difficult to complete if you have a busy working life which uses up all your energy reserves. Both of the detox diets outlined in this *Quick Guide* begin at the weekend to make the initial two-day diet of fruit and water only that bit easier.

Make sure that you have all the healthy ingredients you will need for your diet before you start, and remove from sight any food which is not included in the diet and which you might find too tempting. It is also important to have a relaxed state of mind when on the diet. Do not pick a time when you are generally stressed or are going through some major upheaval in your life, such as moving house. In order to make the diet more enjoyable, make sure that you have plenty of good reading material, music or whatever other non-active pastimes you enjoy, close at hand.

While on either diet it is advisable to take a daily multi-vitamin pill which contains no sugar, yeast or artificial colourings or flavourings, as your body will suddenly be deprived of many of the foods which it is used to, such as bread and dairy products. It is also best to take a daily dose of fish oil or evening primrose oil, because your diet will contain very few essential fatty acids, and none at all in the first two days. Essential fatty acids are found in vegetable and fish oils, and they play a very important role in the function of every cell in your body. These oils can be taken in capsule form. Before you begin either diet, it is important to eat as healthily as possible and have a pre-diet day where you give up all stimulants such as tea, coffee and alcohol, and eat as much raw food as possible. This will make the first day of your detox diet less of a strain.

Side-effects

You will probably experience some side-effects during the process of detoxification in the same way that you get a headache after a night of heavy drinking. A hangover is basically a group of symptoms which are caused by your body's attempt to rid itself of the excessive amount of alcohol which you have given it. Detoxing gives the body a chance to release excess toxins in a similar way. Here are some of the common side-effects you may experience on either diet, some more severe than others:

* Headaches – you will probably experience headaches during the first forty-eight hours of the diet. This is especially true if you are addicted to caffeine. The worse the headache, the higher the level of toxicity. If the headaches are unbearable you may have to drink one cup of black coffee.

* Nausea – you may experience this in the initial forty-eight-hour fast.

* You may feel unusually cold because you are eating less food and therefore will have less energy. To conserve this energy wear as many layers of clothes as you need to keep warm and turn the heating up.

* Constipation – even though you are eating only raw foods, you may experience some constipation while your bowels get used to this new regime.

* Diarrhoea – alternatively, your bowel movements may work overtime to remove all the toxins which your body is trying rapidly to eliminate.

* Skin rashes and pimples – another sign that your body is eliminating toxins.

* Weight-loss – because you are suddenly eating much less food, you will probably lose some weight, but after the first couple of days the rate at which you lose it should slow down. Most people find this a welcome side effect!

—4—

The Detox Diet

The Seven-day Detox Diet

Saturday and Sunday: All detox programmes begin with a period of fasting; you should either have a water-only fast or eat one kind of fruit only. If you can bear it, try to drink as many as eight glasses of mineral water, preferably non-carbonated, daily but not while you are eating the fruit, as this can interfere with your body's digestion. Water is a natural detoxifier which helps to flush out any build-up of toxins inside the system by binding them with the fibre in the fruit and vegetables before they are excreted. Drinking water half an hour before a meal also gives you a temporary sense of fullness which helps prevent hunger pangs. Try to drink mineral water instead of tap water which is full of nitrates, chlorine, aluminium and other unwanted substances. When chosing a mineral water select varieties which have a low sodium and nitrate content. In the same way that you lose your appetite when you are ill, in order for the body to properly rid itself of toxins you need to give your body a rest with a two-day fast. Fasting, far from endangering your health, is actually very beneficial if carried out regularly as it relieves the body of clogged-up toxins, stabilises body weight and helps to prepare the body to utilise nutrients far more effectively.

It is vitally important that you rest during this period, as you will have very little energy, and remember to keep drinking water. If possible, try and eat organic fruit or at least wash any fruit before eating it (see page 9). The fruit should be eaten raw as it contains valuable enzymes that trigger a huge range of chemical reactions within the body. Enzymes also perish when exposed to air and so fruit is best eaten as soon as it has been cut. The nutrient values of fruit also begin to diminish as soon as the fruit is picked. The reason why you should only eat one kind of fruit during this detox diet is that the enzymes in different fruits can interfere with each other, making digestion of them more difficult. However, you can switch to another variety of fruit on the Sunday. You will probably need to have a piece of fruit every hour or so because it does not stay in your stomach for very long. Avoid citrus fruits because they are highly acidic, and bananas because they have a high starch content and, unless eaten when very ripe, are difficult to digest. However, do not fret if bananas are your favourite fruit as they can be eaten in abundance after the initial two days of rapid detox. Bananas are high in fibre and pectin which binds with toxins and helps to remove them from the system.

Here is a list of some of the most effective detoxifying fruits:

* apples – contain useful vitamins, plus malic and tartaric acid which aid digestion, plus apples contain pectin which aids the removal of toxins and prevents protein matter in the intestines from putrefying.

* watermelon – a wonderful detox fruit with a diuretic effect.

* grapes – excellent internal cleansers for the skin, liver, intestines and kidneys, with a high water content.

* mango – this and other tropical fruits contain an enzyme called papain which helps to break down protein wastes in the system. Mangoes also contain high amounts of beta-carotene as well as vitamin C and potassium.

* apricots – a good source of vitamin C, beta-carotene, potassium and calcium.

* pineapple – contains many nutrients including beta-carotene, folic acid, vitamin C, potassium, calcium and magnesium. Pineapple also contains the enzyme bromalin which counteracts bacteria, helps to keep the gut free from infection, and aids the digestion of protein.

Monday and Tuesday: Try to stick to raw food only for the next two days of the detox programme. Both fruit and vegetables are a valuable source of fibre, carbohydrates, minerals, vitamins and enzymes; the only way to ensure that you receive all these nutrients is to eat them raw. Vitamins are especially vulnerable as they tend to be water soluble and are absorbed in the cooking water. If you want cooked vegetables, then it is best to stir-fry them quickly in a little olive oil so that they are lightly cooked, or to lightly steam them in a steamer placed over a saucepan containing a little boiling water. You can also have some boiled short-grain brown rice with one of your daily meals. Raw foods are much easier for your body to digest and, therefore, speed up the elimination of toxins. Choose your meals from menu **A** in the **meal plans** chapter of this *Quick Guide* or create your own, but keep it raw! These menus are designed to outline what sort of foods you should be eating with a few suggested recipes. You can eat foods which are not mentioned in the menus as long as they are in the specified food groups.

Wednesday and Thursday: You can now gradually bring in fish, chicken and shellfish to your diet, and a minimal amount of low-fat dairy produce such as skimmed milk and cottage cheese. Choose any meals from menus **A** and **B** and create some of your own.

Friday: This is the last day of your detox diet. You can eat wheat in the form of wholemeal bread (this is probably one of the most difficult things you had to live without, but don't compensate for its absence in one day!). You can also eat red meat and full-fat dairy foods if you wish, but only one or the other and in minimal amounts, as both foods are very high in saturated fat. Choose any of the meals from menus **A**, **B** and **C** or create your own.

The Twenty-one-day Detox Diet

This longer diet is designed to allow your body to detox at a steadier, more gradual pace and it is ideal for those who have a considerably poor diet or are perhaps recovering from a drawn-out illness. It should start a steady release of all toxins which have built up in your system and will hopefully help you establish healthier eating patterns for the future. The diet starts at the weekend with a water and fruit fast, then in Week 1 you can move on to other raw foods; in Week 2 you can start to eat fish, chicken and limited low-fat dairy products; and finally in Week 3 you can gradually introduce, in small amounts, other dairy products, wheat products and red meat. By this time your taste buds and whole body will have adapted to this healthy eating regime, and you will probably not want to go back to eating processed foods and high-fat dairy products.

Saturday and Sunday: Drink plenty of still mineral water, aiming for about eight glasses a day, and as much of one type of fruit as you want. To find out which fruits are best suited to this detox programme see the paragraph at the beginning of the seven-day diet outline (see page 36).

Week 1 Monday–Sunday: Try to stick to raw food only and remember that this does not just mean fruit and vegetables. There are a wide variety of nuts and seeds to choose from which are packed with protein and taste great (see the section on nuts and seeds on page 00). If you can't bear the thought of another raw meal, then you can have cooked wholegrains such as brown rice and steamed or stir-fried vegetables. Choose anything from menu **A** in the **meal plans** chapter of this *Quick Guide* or create your own meals.

Week 2 Monday–Sunday: You can now start eating chicken and other white meat, preferably free-range, eggs, fish and only very low-fat dairy products such as skimmed milk and low-fat cottage cheese. However, these foods should only be eaten in limited amounts and the bulk of your diet should continue to be raw fruit and vegetables. Choose any of the meals from menu **A** and **B** in the **meal plans** chapter and remember to keep drinking mineral water.

Week 3 Monday–Friday: Most toxins should now have been eliminated from your body so you can start to introduce wheat products, red meat and dairy products to your diet in moderation. Do not introduce more than one of these food types each day. Bring in wheat products at the beginning of the week, red meat mid-week and dairy products last at the end of the week. After three weeks of healthy eating you should feel 100 percent healthier and fitter and full of vitality. Choose any meals from menus **A**, **B** and **C** or create your own.

Try not to slip back into bad habits of eating lots of fatty cheeses, processed foods and drinking several cups of coffee as soon as the detox diet is over, as this will start to undo all the good work you have done. Continue to drink plenty of pure water, eat lots of fruit and vegetables and drink alcohol in moderation.

—— 5 ——
Meal Plans

Menu A

Eat mostly raw food, no dairy products (except live yoghurt), meat, fish, or wheat products, and drink plenty of mineral water.

Breakfast:

* Have a cup of hot water with a slice of lemon as a substitute for your usual cup of tea or coffee; the lemon juice will stimulate the bowels and help to eliminate toxins. Or have a herbal tea. (These will be discussed separately – see page 62.)

* Have a meal of fruit, perhaps a fruit salad (no bananas) with some added sliced almonds or other nuts and mixed with low-fat live yoghurt.

* If you find it difficult to eat anything in the morning, then make a juice out of fresh fruit or vegetables. Most juices in cartons are processed and many have added sugar. Many are made from frozen, devitalised fruit concentrate and tap water. Drinking *fresh* vegetable and fruit juices is an easy way to get a large amount of concentrated nutritional goodness without having to eat pounds of the actual food. Juice puts the digestive system under less strain than the whole fruit or vegetable does because the juicing process removes

most of the fibre. To make the most of juicing you really need an electronic juicer as doing it by hand is a laborious process. Choose your fruits/vegetables from the following list: apples, carrot, celery, cucumber, grapes, grapefruit, mango, melon, orange, papaya, peach, pear, pineapple, strawberry, and watermelon.

Lunch and dinner:

* A large salad from any raw vegetables. The following are particularly suited to a detox diet: artichoke, asparagus, beetroot, bean sprouts, cabbage, carrot, cauliflower, celeriac, celery, chicory, Chinese leaves, chives, cress, cucumber, green beans, green peas, kale, lollo rosso, mange-tout, onions, peppers, radish, spring greens, sweetcorn and watercress. Avoid tomatoes, spinach, rhubarb and sorrel because they contain large amounts of oxalic acid which can be irritating to the gut. Make a salad dressing out of fresh herbs (see the herbs section on page 62 of this *Quick Guide*) and olive oil with a squeeze of lemon juice.

* Baked potato with cottage cheese or tzatziki (made from low-fat live yoghurt, thinly sliced cucumber, crushed garlic with fresh or dried mint and black pepper) and a small mixed salad.

* A mixture of stir-fried or steamed vegetables mixed with a combination of pulses (such as soya protein, tofu or chick peas), with a cup of boiled short-grain brown rice.

* You can snack on any unsalted nuts, seeds or fruit (including bananas). Both nuts and seeds are very

nutritious. They are rich in vitamin E and many minerals including zinc and iron, and are packed with protein.

∗ Brown rice and hazelnut salad is a delicious detox meal made with brown rice, unsalted hazelnuts, currants, sunflower seeds, spring onions, dark lettuce and some freshly chopped parsley.

RECIPES

Stuffed red peppers
Serves 1
To make the stuffing, preheat the oven to 190°C (375°F, gas mark 5). Then fry half a chopped onion in olive oil. Add some grated carrot and about 50g (2oz) of short-grain brown rice to the pan. Pour in 200ml (1/4 pint) of vegetable or chicken stock and add some peas, raisins, thyme, salt and pepper. Prepare a couple of peppers by removing the stalk and seeds and then bake them in the oven for 15–20 minutes. Remove from the oven and stuff with the rice mixture.

Asparagus and mushroom risotto
Serves 2
Lightly toast 100g (4oz) of brown rice and then add 475ml (16fl oz) of water, one chopped onion and a few strands of saffron (optional). Bring to the boil, cover and simmer for 20 minutes.

Meanwhile, chop 100g (4oz) asparagus into short lengths, reserving the tips for garnish. After the 20 minutes' cooking time add the lengths of asparagus and simmer for another 10–15 minutes until the rice is soft.

In a separate pan, gently heat 2 teaspoons of cold-pressed olive oil and lightly sauté the asparagus tips. Remove from the

pan and drain on kitchen paper. Stir 100g (4oz) chopped mushrooms and parsley into the cooked rice mixture. Season with
black pepper, stir in a little lemon juice and serve garnished with
the asparagus tips.

Millet mash
Serves 3–4
Heat 1 teaspoon of sesame or cold-pressed olive oil and gently
fry a chopped onion until transparent. Stir in 1 tablespoon of
tamari sauce and add 175–225g (6–8oz) of cauliflower or broc-
coli, cut into florets, 200g (7oz) of millet and 600ml (1 pint) of
water. Bring to the boil briefly, then cover and simmer until
soft. Mash until smooth and serve with chopped tomatoes and
fresh parsley.

Menu B

You can now gradually introduce certain low-fat dairy produce
such as cottage cheese, skimmed milk and plain live yoghurt, as
well as chicken and fish, into your diet. Drink plenty of mineral
water.

Breakfast:

* Start the day as usual with a cup of hot water and
  lemon or a herbal tea.

* Bircher muesli – you can make this easily from mixing
  together rolled oats, low-fat live yoghurt, cold water,
  grated lemon rind, freshly grated apple, soft fruit such
  as strawberries and hazelnuts or almonds.

* ACE compote is my own recipe for an ideal fast-food

breakfast which is high in the antioxidant vitamins A (in the form of beta-carotene), C and E, and it is prepared the night before. To make this, soak a selection of dried fruit (which should be unsulphured) in water overnight with some allspice and cinnamon. In the morning add some low-fat live yoghurt to the mixture with some chopped almonds.

* Bran flakes with skimmed milk.

* Hot bulgar breakfast – gently heat a little virgin olive oil in a saucepan and add 40g (1½ oz) of bulgar wheat, 25g (1 oz) of sesame seeds and 25g of wheatgerm, and sauté until lightly browned. Add 150ml (¼ pint) of water and stir in 6g (½ oz) of chopped dried apricots. Cover and simmer for about 25 minutes or until the bulgar is fluffy and the water has been absorbed. Add some chopped nuts to taste.

* Porridge made with rolled oats and skimmed milk with some added fresh or stewed fruit.

Lunch and dinner:

* Any of the meals from menu **A**.

* A poached or boiled egg with a salad or steamed vegetables.

* Roast chicken with the skin removed, potatoes (with the skin on) and steamed vegetables or salad.

* Grilled, steamed or poached fish with potatoes, steamed vegetables or salad.

* Salad Niçoise made with lettuce, tomato, onion,
  cucumber, tuna (canned in olive or soya oil), anchovies
  and hard-boiled eggs.

* Fish risotto – grill some oily fish (eg mackerel or
  herring) and flake into large pieces. Fry some onion in
  olive oil then add the fish, some cooked brown rice and
  some peas. Stir continuously for about 3 minutes and
  then serve with chopped fresh basil or parsley.

* Brown pasta, with tomato sauce and clams or mussels.
  You can use tinned clams or mussels in brine. Make a
  tomato sauce with fresh or tinned tomatoes, chopped
  onion, garlic, fresh basil and black pepper.

* Try using marinated tofu as a meat substitute. It can be
  added to many sauces and is a much healthier low-fat
  option.

RECIPES

Seafood spears
Serves 4
Make a marinade from 4 tablespoons of unrefined sunflower
and safflower oil, the juice of 1 lemon, 1 tablespoon of tamari
sauce, 1 tablespoon of fresh chopped parsley and some freshly
ground black pepper. Then blanch 8 shallots, or 2 large onions,
for 1 minute in boiling water. Cut 750g (1¹/₂ lbs) of fresh or
frozen fish (ideally cod, tuna or salmon) into chunks and thread
together 8 scallops or prawns, shallots or onions, half a chopped
red pepper, half a green pepper and 2 thinly sliced courgettes on
to wooden or metal skewers. Brush with the marinade and place
under a medium heat grill and cook for about 5 minutes
(depending upon the fish). Turn the kebabs twice, brushing

them with the marinade as they cook. Serve on a bed of brown rice and garnish with parsley before serving.

Prawn kebabs with herb dressing
Serves 2
Thread 12 king-sized prawns, 8 button mushrooms and 1 sliced courgette on to metal or wooden skewers and place in a shallow dish. To make the herb dressing, mix together 4 tablespoons of cold-pressed olive oil or refined sunflower oil, 1 clove of garlic, peeled and crushed, the juice of 1 lemon and a sprig each of basil, parsley and tarragon, finely chopped. Pour dressing over the kebabs and leave to marinate for 30 minutes, turning occasionally. Place under a medium grill and cook for about 3 minutes, basting and turning the kebabs as they cook.

Tofu and onion flan
Serves 4
Preheat the oven to 200°C (400°F, gas mark 6). To make the pastry mix together 100g (4oz) of buckwheat flour and 25g (1oz) poppy seeds in a food processor, and slowly dribble in 2 tablespoons of unrefined walnut or hazelnut oil. Add just enough of 50ml (2fl oz) of ice cold water to enable the dough to form a ball around the blade. Put the dough in a bowl, cover with a cloth and place in the fridge for 30 minutes. For the filling, heat 1 teaspoon of olive oil and fry 550g (16oz) of chopped onions until transparent. Place 225g (8oz) of firm silken tofu in the food processor and blend until smooth and the consistency of double cream. Add 150ml (1/4pint) soya milk, 2 teaspoons of mustard, 2 (size 3) free-range eggs and some freshly ground black pepper – and blend again. Roll out the pastry and use to line a 20cm (8 inch) flan dish. Bake blind for 10 minutes. Then reduce the temperature to 160°C (325°F, gas mark 3). Arrange the onions in the pastry case and pour over the tofu mixture. Bake for 45 minutes or until set and turning golden brown.

Menu C

You can eat any of the foods in menus **A** and **B** and now you can also add dairy, wheat, and red meat products to your diet, but keep them to a minimum. You must still avoid all toxic stimulents such as tea, coffee and alcohol and remember to drink plenty of mineral water.

Breakfast:
You should try to stick to the raw breakfasts in menus **A** and **B** but if you really need a change you can have some wholemeal toast and sunflower or soya margarine.

Lunch and dinner:

* Greek salad made with feta cheese, peppers, cucumber, onion, tomatoes and olives.

* Vegetable or chicken soup with a wholemeal roll spread with sunflower or soya margarine.

RECIPES

Spaghetti bolognese
Serve this classic Italian sauce with brown, wholewheat or spelt pasta (made from an ancient grain of wheat – *Triticum spelta* – which is easier to digest). To make the bolognese sauce, fry some chopped onion and garlic in a little olive oil and add some lean minced lamb. Once the mince is browned add chopped tomatoes, mushrooms and peppers, oregano and basil and simmer for 20–25 minutes. You can add some freshly grated Parmesan cheese before serving.

Spinach and macaroni pie
Serves 4

Preheat the oven to 190°C (375°F, gas mark 5). Cook 300g (11oz) of dried wholewheat macaroni following the instructions on the packet. Rinse in cold water and drain. Wash 450g (1lb) of fresh spinach and chop it into small pieces. Cook it in boiling water for 2–3 minutes. Place the spinach in a large mixing bowl and add 50ml (2fl oz) of skimmed milk, a chopped medium-sized onion, 3 crushed garlic cloves, and some grated ginger root to season. Stir in the cooked macaroni and transfer to a baking dish. Mix together 100g (4oz) of wholewheat bread-crumbs, 50g (2oz) of Parmesan cheese and 25g (1oz) of sesame seeds. Sprinkle this mixture over the macaroni mixture and bake in the oven for 20–25 minutes or until the breadcrumb topping is crisp and golden.

Chicken with lemon

Preheat the oven to 220°C (425°F, gas mark 7). Stuff a small free-range chicken with some lemon peel, an onion, a sprig of tarragon, 25g (1oz) of butter, some freshly ground black pepper and a little salt.

Squeeze the juice of one lemon and coat the outside of the chicken with it, adding a little salt and pepper. Place the chicken on parchment baking paper with a thin covering of olive oil and smear a little more olive oil on to the breast and legs. Bring up the sides of the baking paper to form a loose parcel and wrap this in an outer sheet of foil.

Place in the oven to roast for about an hour. Halfway through cooking, remove the chicken from the oven and baste thoroughly. Open the top of the parcel for the last 10 minutes, allowing the breast to brown. Serve with a mixed salad.

Spiced bananas
Serves 2

Peel and slice 2 ripe bananas and place in individual serving bowls. In a small saucepan melt 50g (2oz) of butter or soya margarine, and stir in half a tablespoon of clear honey and 1 teaspoon of allspice. Pour over the bananas and serve immediately.

This recipe works well with pears too.

6

Detox Diet Boosters

Nuts and Seeds

Nuts and seeds are very nutritious, they are rich in vitamin E and many minerals including zinc and iron. Although relatively high in calories, nuts are an excellent protein-packed alternative to high-fat cheese and meat. All nuts should be eaten raw and as fresh as possible as they turn rancid when exposed to heat or light. However, be aware that nuts are common food allergens. All processed, dry-roasted or salted nuts should be avoided in this detox programme. Seeds too are a rich source of concentrated goodness, particularly sprouted alfalfa seeds which taste great in salads.

NUTS

Almonds – these nuts are a good source of protein and several important minerals including zinc and iron. They also contain essential fatty acids.

Brazils – they are a useful source of the essential amino acid methionine and are best eaten as a fast-food snack or mixed with other types of nuts in a salad.

Hazelnuts – all nuts contain polyunsaturated fat, but hazelnuts have the lowest amount. Like almonds, they are also rich in vitamin E which fights free-radicals, the destructive particles that damage cells.

Peanuts – these are not really nuts at all but belong to the same legume family as the soya bean. They are especially rich in protein, iron, vitamin E and B vitamins (notably folic acid). However, all legumes can be hard to digest and peanuts are no exception.

Walnuts – these are the best nuts for a great-tasting detox salad and are an essential ingredient of the famous Waldorf salad which combines walnuts, chopped apple and crunchy celery.

SEEDS

Alfalfa seeds – when these precious seeds are sprouted their vitamin content increases by up to 700 percent! The sprouts are one of the few vegetables to contain vitamin B12, which is most common in meat, so all vegetarians should make these seeds an integral part of their diet. You can sprout alfalfa seeds at home by sprinkling them on damp blotting paper, but they can be bought already sprouted from good health food shops. Alfalfa sprouts act as a mild diuretic and intestinal cleanser and are therefore a perfect part of any detox diet.

Pumpkin seeds – Hungarians have claimed that these seeds can improve your sex life and it must be due to the high zinc content. Pumpkin seeds also contain iron, calcium and many B vitamins. They make an excellent addition to salads and are great to snack on too.

Sesame seeds – these seeds are packed with calcium and protein as well as iron and zinc. They also contain useful amounts of vitamin E and lecithin which are both essential for strong skin. Vitamin E destroys free-radicals and lecithin is a fatty substance which locks moisture into the skin, preventing dry skin and fighting premature ageing. More importantly, sesame seeds are a particularly good source of one of the eight essential amino acids called methionine. This is needed for healthy kidney functioning which is essential to detoxing. Sesame seeds are very versatile and can be added to virtually any recipe.

Sunflower seeds – in Russia millions survived a famine by living on sunflower seeds and virtually nothing else for months on end, so you should certainly be able to survive a brief detox diet if you eat plenty of these. They have high levels of vitamins, minerals, fibre, essential fatty acids, protein and amino acids. Sunflower seeds also contain pectin which helps prevent lead poisoning from car exhausts, and also helps to remove toxic wastes from the body by combining with them and enabling them to be excreted. Almost half the sunflower seed is taken up with polyunsaturates, the beneficial fats that keep our cholesterol levels in check and prevent our arteries from becoming clogged. The seeds taste great in salads and you can cook foods in sunflower oil as long as it is unrefined. Both the seeds and unrefined sunflower oil can be bought from health food shops.

Both nuts and seeds are very versatile and can be added to many meals, especially salads, or just eaten on their own as snacks. They can also be combined in delicious recipes like hummus. This Greek delicacy is cheap and simple to make and it is a great filling for sandwiches or baked potatoes, or as a dip for vegetables. Hummus can be kept for a few days when stored in the fridge. Here is a recipe for 2–4 people.

HUMMUS

Soak 50g (2oz) of chick peas overnight in cold water, or for 2 hours in boiling water, then cook for 4 hours. Then place the cooked chick peas, juice of 1 lemon, 2 cloves of garlic (crushed), 1 tablespoon of olive oil, 1 tablespoon of tahini (sesame seed paste) and 50ml (2fl oz) of water (optional) in a food processor and blend until smooth. If you don't have a food processor, then place all the ingredients into a large mixing bowl and pound with a potato masher, if necessary adding a little water to make the mixture smooth. Serve garnished with parsley and pine nuts.

Whole Grains

Delicious and nutritious grains and cereals safely boost our fibre intake and increase our protein and mineral supplies. Two daily servings of these complex carbohydrates also give the body a slow, sustained release of energy throughout the day, regulate blood sugar levels and reduce cravings for sweet and fatty foods. A daily portion of oat bran has even been found to regulate insulin production and be helpful to diabetics.

It is important to avoid wheat on a detox diet, which means no pasta and bread, even if it is wholemeal. This is because wheat bran interferes with the absorption of some of our most important nutrients such as iron, calcium and magnesium, and can irritate the sensitive lining of the intestines. Wheat also contains gluten which can block the small intestine. Some people are particularly intolerant to gluten and the symptoms of this include diarrhoea, anaemia due to poor iron absorption, tiredness and recurrent mouth ulcers. Gluten can also cause a skin reaction called *dermatitis herpetiformis* which is recognised by an itchy red rash or tiny sore blisters just beneath the surface of the skin.

Irritable bowel syndrome is just one of the many modern diseases triggered by a lethal mixture of poor diet and stress. Sufferers are usually advised to switch from wheat to gluten-free grains and often find that their symptoms of bloating, constipation or diarrhoea disappear.

Rices, millet, buckwheat, barley and quinoa are all gluten-free whole grains which are very quick and simple to cook. All grains must be washed by rinsing them under a running tap in a sieve.

Barley – this nutritious whole grain has high levels of iron, calcium, potassium and B vitamins and it has soothing properties on the stomach, digestive and urinary tracts. Unrefined barley, known as pot barley, is coated in a thin layer of nutritious barley bran. It should be soaked overnight before using, but keep the soaking water for cooking as it will contain important vitamins. It takes about an hour to cook pot barley and it is a delicious addition to rice dishes. Barley water is an excellent internal tonic and kidney cleanser and can be used to treat stomach ulcers, cystitis and constipation. To make this, pour 1½ pints (900ml) of water over 1oz (30g) wholegrain barley (not pearl barley) and boil until the quantity is reduced by half. Then sweeten with a little honey or apple juice.

Buckwheat – this is the favourite food of healthy and long-living Buddhist monks. As part of the *Kaiho-gyo* ritual of prayer for the attainment of higher spiritual powers, the monks undertake a 100-day fast when they eat nothing but buckwheat. Buckwheat is totally gluten-free and nothing like common wheat. It is actually a seed from a dock-like plant and contains B vitamins, potassium, magnesium and iron. Buckwheat grouts can be washed and cooked in the same way as rice, and buckwheat flour can be substituted for wheat flour in baking and to thicken soups and sauces.

Cornflour – this is a great gluten-free thickener for soups and sauces.

Millet – this is the gluten-free seed of a grass native to Asia (it is not just budgie fodder!). It is a complete protein, which means that it contains all eight essential amino acids. It also contains more iron than other cereals and is an excellent source of calcium. It also contains silica which is a skin-cleansing, strengthening and healing agent. It can be cooked as an alternative to rice, but 'crack' the tiny seeds first by frying them in a little olive oil. This helps them to absorb enough water to become soft.

Oats – these contain vitamins B and E as well as healthy polyunsaturates. They are also rich in calcium, potassium and magnesium and can be made into two breakfast dishes – porridge and muesli.

Quinoa – this is pronounced 'keenowa' and it is a tiny, golden grain similar to millet. It contains twice as much protein as other grains and it is a source of both essential fatty acids and amino acids. Typically, a single serving supplies over 9g of protein and almost all the amino acids. It has a very bland flavour but it can be mixed with other grains.

Rice – there are over 7,000 varieties of rice including those that are organically grown. All types of rice are easily digested and highly unlikely to cause any allergy problems. Puffed rice makes a good breakfast cereal (you can find sugar-free, organically grown varieties in health food shops) and rice cakes are tasty low-calorie snacks. All rices and rice products are gluten-free.

Rye – rye has a similar composition to wheat but has a low-gluten content. Black rye bread with rye flour is a delicious alternative to your usual loaf, and toasts well. Rye crispbreads and crackers are also easy to find in the supermarket and make an interesting change to wheat-based varieties. Rye flour can also be mixed with wheat flour for home baking.

Wheat – this is Britain's most important crop and, not surprisingly, our diet is dominated by it. There are over 30,000 varieties which belong to two main species; these are *Triticum aestivum* used for bread baking, and a harder wheat called *Triticum durum* used for making pasta and semolina. Unfortunately, wheat and all its products have a high gluten content (even the wholemeal varieties) and so it is worthwhile trying a period of wheat-free eating every once in a while.

Acidity and Alkalinity

A body that is overloaded with toxins tends to have a high level of acidity as the majority of stored wastes are acidic. The detox diet outlined in this *Quick Guide* should restore your body's natural pH (level of acidity) as it includes mostly fresh fruit and vegetables which are alkali-forming. All animal proteins such as meat, fish, poultry and eggs are acidic as are most grains, bread and cereals. A balanced diet should generally consist of only 20 percent acid-forming food and 80 percent alkali-forming food. Study the table below to find out those which are acid-forming and those which are alkali-forming.

Food Combining

This method of eating also promotes better digestion and so is useful when following any detox regime. It is based on the principle that many fats and carbohydrates (particularly refined carbohydrates such as white bread and pasta, sugary products, and processed foods), when eaten with a concentrated form of protein (meat, fish and cheese), slow down the digestion of protein and so build up waste. It is, therefore, best not to combine these foods while on the detox programme. This of

Acid-forming foods	Alkali-forming foods
barley	almonds
beans	brazil nuts
bread	chestnuts
breakfast cereals	fruit
buckwheat	hazelnuts
cashew nuts	milk
cheese	millet
chick peas	pine kernels
eggs	vegetables
fish	
flour	
game	
meat	
oats	
peanuts	
pecan nuts	
poultry	
rice	
sugar	
walnuts	
wheat	

course means giving up very traditional meals such as pies, quiches, many pasta dishes and even most sandwiches. Any cooked meals you have should involve unrefined carbohydrates, such as brown rice, potatoes and other whole grains, with steamed or stir-fried vegetables. This will give you the maximum amount of nutrition you can get from cooked food, and it will minimise any build-up of waste. Here are some basic guidelines as to how to make food combining part of your detox programme:

* Try to have fruit on its own for breakfast as your body is most actively detoxing between midnight and midday and what you eat in the morning is crucial to its success.

* Don't eat a concentrated starch food (pasta, rice, bread, potatoes and bananas) with a concentrated protein food (meat, poultry, fish, eggs and cheese).

* Leave at least four hours between a starch meal and a protein meal.

* Make one of your daily meals a huge raw salad as all the fibre, vitamins and minerals are a valuable part of any detoxing diet.

* Eliminate all processed foods from your diet.

* Chew every mouthful properly!

The Way to Chew

To get the most from your food, it is best to eat in a relaxed environment where you can sit down and savour every mouthful properly. Many of us lead such busy lives that we end up eating a sandwich while on the run. Few people realise how important it is to chew every mouthful thoroughly to enable our body to digest the food properly. When we chew something, we decrease the size of food particles; this increases the food's surface area, making it easier for enzymes to do their job of breaking down the food. This breaking-down process enables our bodies to utilise all the nutrients in the food without building up excessive wastes. Chewing also produces salivary amylase enzymes which digest carbohydrates. If there is a lot of fat in your diet, this will inhibit the digestive process because it inhibits the secretion of gastric acid and the enzyme pepsin in the stomach. This results in food not being digested properly, limiting the amount of nutrients you get from the food and creating a build-up of waste.

A friend once told me how the nuns in her convent school used to make the pupils chew each mouthful of food fifteen times. This seemed like another cruel, pointless rule at the time, but now she realises how important proper chewing is in order for us to digest our food fully.

7

Herbs and Supplements

Sea Vegetables

All seaweeds are rich in the minerals which your body needs in order for its metabolic processes to function properly. Some of these minerals are only needed by the body in minute amounts, but because our normal food sources have been depleted of much of their nutritional value due to modern farming methods and pollution, we need to get certain nutrients elsewhere. Some sea plants are rich in special forms of fibre called alginates which have the ability to bind and remove heavy metals from the body. They are also rich in organic iodine which tends to stimulate metabolic processes. Kelp can be bought in supplement form, but make sure that it has been collected from unpolluted waters and then 'atomised' or broken into very fine particles. This process of atomisation is very important because seaweeds tend to have very hard cell walls and these walls need to be exploded to allow our bodies access to their mineral content.

SPIRULINA

This is a particularly special form of blue-green algae and it grows in abundance in warm fresh water. It was the staple food of the Aztecs of Mexico and it is an astonishing source of protein. It is possibly the most antioxidant and nutritious plant on this earth and it contains all eight essential amino acids plus ten other amino acids. These amino acids are superior to those found in meat and eggs as they are alkaline rather than acidic. While your body is detoxing it is trying to eliminate stored wastes which are generally acidic, so the alkaline form of amino acids is easier for the body to digest. Amino acids are very important in terms of building new cells, tissues, hormones and body enzymes. Spirulina is also nature's richest source of vitamin B12 (which prevents us from developing anaemia), and of iron. It contains fifty-eight times more iron than raw spinach.

Spirulina is particularly beneficial for those on a detox programme as it contains virtually every antioxidant known to man including the ACE vitamins A, C and E. In fact, it contains three times more vitamin E than wheatgerm, and a startling twenty-eight times more beta-carotene (the precursor to vitamin A) than raw carrots. Spirulina also contains vitamins C, B1, B5 and B6 as well as the minerals zinc, manganese and copper and the trace element selenium.

This unbelievable algae is also a rare source of the essential fatty acid GLA (gamma-linolenic acid) which helps to form new cell walls. If the cell walls are not properly formed, cell metabolism and the elimination of wastes can be affected. Spirulina is three times richer in GLA than evening primrose oil.

Herbs and Spices

Many herbs have a cleansing effect on the body and can be easily added to salads or drunk in the form of herbal teas as part of this detox programme. Many herbs are natural diuretics and these are better than chemical diuretics which deplete the body of potassium. All diuretic herbs contain potassium which bypasses this problem. Diuretics provoke an increase in the flow of urine and this is one way of ridding the body of toxins. Dandelion leaves, parsley, celery, asparagus, horsetail and juniper are particularly good herbal diuretics. Other herbs boost detoxification through the skin by encouraging perspiration, such as ginger and peppermint.

Formulations of many detoxifying herbs are available in pill or capsule form, but it is better to eat the natural plants, where available, as these tend to be high in a variety of different vitamins and minerals.

Aloe vera – this versatile herb has an impressive history of use since the time of the Ancient Egyptians. It can be used both externally, to soothe burns and skin irritations, and internally to ease constipation. Aloe vera has a calming effect on the stomach and eases digestion. It is particularly helpful in the digestion of proteins. There are many skin creams available containing aloe vera, and supplements which are taken internally can also be bought from good health food shops.

Burdock – this was used in the past as a medicinal herb and as a flavouring for the drink dandelion and burdock. Both dandelion and burdock are excellent detox herbs. Burdock has a cleansing effect on body tissue and acts as a mild diuretic and laxative. You can make a tea using 1–2g of the dried herb.

Camomile – this flower has a long history of use as a domestic remedy for indigestion and as a mild laxative. Camomile tea can be bought easily and this is a relaxing herbal tea to have before going to bed.

Capsicums – cayenne pepper can be added to cooked sauces to add a bit of spice and it is also a counter-irritant and should protect your stomach from reacting badly to any food.

Caraway – caraway has a characteristic flavour similar to that of dill and is used in carminative mixtures such as gripe water. It has a soothing action on the gut and eases any flatulence (wind). The dried seeds are widely available and can be added to sauces.

Cardamom – cardamom seeds are a common ingredient of vegetable curries and they help to stimulate digestion and circulation, as well as having a general carminative effect.

Cinnamon – this spice has been used for many years to treat nausea, vomiting, diarrhoea and colds. It is now frequently used to flavour apple pies and other cooked fruits and it has a carminative effect on the stomach as well as being a delicious and warming digestive tonic.

Coriander – This digestive aid is wonderfully aromatic and is used in spices and curries throughout the world. Coriander seeds stimulate the appetite and relieve colic and flatulence.

Dandelion – this is a very good diuretic and it is also high in potassium which can replace that which is lost in the diuretic process. It is also a very good digestive tonic and can be bought as a herbal tea. Dandelion also contains the antioxidant beta-carotene. (See also Burdock.)

Fennel – this is another herb with a carminative action on the body. It tastes like aniseed and the fresh herb can be chopped and added to salads. Fennel stimulates circulation and is a good diuretic. It can also be bought in health food shops as a delicious herbal tea.

Garlic – cloves of garlic are antiviral especially when it comes to the digestive system. There is some evidence which suggests that garlic attacks viruses while leaving friendly micro-organisms unharmed. It is also an excellent blood cleanser and can reduce blood pressure. Garlic contains antiseptic substances which can help clear mucus conditions and bronchitis. Try and eat at least one clove of garlic a day, which is not difficult as it tastes great in virtually every savoury dish. You can eat some fresh parsley afterwards to remove the smell, but if you can't bear to eat garlic, then you can buy odourless garlic capsules in chemists or health food shops.

Ginger – the root of the ginger plant is an excellent carminative and has been used for centuries to prevent sea sickness and other forms of motion sickness. It can be chopped up and added to stir-fries to create a lovely spicy flavour.

Hyssop – this is a great herb for detoxifying the lungs. It has a slightly bitter aroma and has been used medically as a stimulant in the treatment of asthma and bronchitis. It also has an anti-inflammatory activity. Mix a few drops of hyssop essential oil with some hot water in a bath or a bowl and inhale the aroma to clear the lungs.

Juniper – the oil present in juniper berries acts as a wonderful carminative and it is also often used to flavour meat and pâtés. Juniper berries are a natural diuretic, although in large doses they can harm the kidneys. They also boost the elimination of acid and act as a general digestive tonic. Herbalists recommend taking one gram of the dried berries a day to feel the diuretic effect. Do not take a mixture of many diuretic herbs each day as this will be too much for your system to cope with.
  Caution: Do not use juniper if you have a kidney infection or are pregnant.

Lemon – lemons are a wonderful detox fruit and they have a surprisingly low level of acid. Lemon is a good diuretic and a slice of lemon in hot water drunk when you wake up and before you go to sleep will encourage the elimination of toxins.

Parsley – this common kitchen herb can be used fresh to garnish almost anything and it tastes great in salads. Few people are aware that it is also a strong diuretic as well as a carminative and digestive tonic. It is also very nutritious with large quantities of vitamins A and E, iron, calcium, phosphorus and manganese. Parsley is particularly good at removing heavy metals such as lead from the body.

Peppermint – peppermint oil contains menthol and it is widely used as a carminative. It is generally good for nervous bowel, flatulence and colic, all of which interfere with the body's ability to eliminate toxins. Peppermint tea is delicious and can be widely bought.

Rosemary – this culinary herb is mainly used to flavour savoury meat dishes. It stimulates circulation and it has a relaxing and restorative effect on the nervous system. Many of us have very sluggish circulation due to exposure to toxins and herbalists may treat this with 1–4g of dried rosemary or the equivalent taken in capsule form.

Thyme – this is a particularly savoury herb which is mainly used in stuffings. It is a relaxing expectorant which will ease up any build-up of mucus in the throat and lungs. It is also a calming digestive tonic and good if you are having digestive problems or are feeling very constipated. Thyme tea can be made by infusing 1–4g of the dried herb which may then be sweetened with honey.

—— 8 ——
Lymphatic Drainage

To benefit fully from a detox programme, your body's organs of elimination need to be boosted in other ways than just through diet alone. This complex process of detoxification involving many of the body's organs may be severely clogged up with toxins, and will need the combination of a toxin-free diet and stimulation of the lymphatic drainage system. As we have seen, the lymph carries toxins through the body to a place where they can be eliminated by an organ of detoxification, like a waste disposal system. Few people realise the importance of this system but, without it, the kidneys, the bowels, the skin, and the lungs would not be able to do their jobs properly. Its waste-eliminating functions are so vital that without them we would die in just twenty-four hours. The lymphatic system is also a major route for the absorption of nutrients from the digestive system into the tissues, and an important carrier of immune cells which protect your body from infection and prevent degenerative ageing. The lymphatic drainage system can be boosted by daily skin brushing and self-massage.

Skin Brushing

This was previously frowned upon as an activity for those with masochistic tendencies, but now most health practitioners perceive it as something very beneficial. Daily skin brushing removes the dead skin from your pores, allowing them to breathe and absorb any detoxifying lotions and essential oils which you may wish to apply afterwards. More importantly, it leaves the pores unblocked so that the skin can eliminate toxins effectively through them. The skin is the largest eliminative organ, and if it cannot function properly, then this puts enormous pressure on the other eliminative organs in the body such as the bowels, lungs and kidneys. Few people are aware of the extent to which their pores are blocked by dead skin cells, sebum, sweat, bacteria and pollutants. A quick wash with soap and water may not unblock clogged pores – your skin needs to be brushed with a coarse, bristle brush. Try brushing your skin in direct sunlight and you will see hundreds of tiny flakes of dead skin fly away from your body.

Body brushing also stimulates blood flow and gets oxygen to all the parts of the body. It involves long, relatively hard brush strokes towards the heart and this greatly stimulates circulation and the lymphatic drainage system. However, this can not be carried out with a soft bath brush or loofah. There is only one kind of brush which can stimulate the lymphatic system effectively. This is a brush made from natural fibres which has a wooden base and a detachable long wooden handle which makes brushing the hard-to-reach areas of your back much easier. It is relatively cheap and can be bought from most good chemists. You should begin the skin brushing at the same time that you start the detox diet and continue to spend five minutes each day on this important detox activity. Try to do it every day for a couple of weeks, then limit it to a couple of days a week, varying the days, so as to 'surprise' your skin. This should ensure that your skin does not get so used to the brushing sensation that it loses its beneficial effects. Skin brushing will feel odd at first and you probably will not be able to apply much pressure at the beginning. However, most people grow to enjoy the tingling sensation as body brushing revitalises the skin after a while, and feel that it is as much a part of their daily routine as brushing their teeth.

Daily skin brushing will leave your skin feeling revitalised and smoother looking. It is great to do it as soon as you get up in the morning before washing, as this will really wake you up and spur your body into action. You should start by brushing your fingers and hands, brushing between each finger and then the palm and the top of each hand. Continue to brush in long strokes up your arms to just above your elbow, and brush upwards from the same point above the elbow to your shoulder. Always use long, firm strokes in the direction of the heart. Then go on to brush from your toes and the soles of your feet up your legs to your knees, and then from your knees up over each thigh. This is easier to do with the foot of the leg you are brushing resting on a chair or on the side of the bath. Repeat each stroke a few times until you feel that your circulation has really been stimulated (you should experience an invigorating tingling sensation). Then brush your buttocks in long circular movements from the outside inwards towards the inner thigh where the lymph glands are located. Go on to brush upwards the lower part of your back and when you have finished brushing the lower half of your body, brush downwards from the neck over your chest and upper back. If you can bear it, brush in small, gentle strokes inside the armpits where you also have lymph glands. When brushing and massaging these areas you are stimulating the lymphatic drainage system directly.

After body brushing regularly for a couple of weeks, you should notice an improvement in the tone of your skin. Don't brush skin which is broken or irritated in any way. You can wash the brush every couple of weeks in warm water, using a natural soap. Rinse it with cold water and shake dry or leave it in a warm place, such as an airing cupboard, to thoroughly dry out.

Always brush your body using long, firm strokes in the direction of the heart.

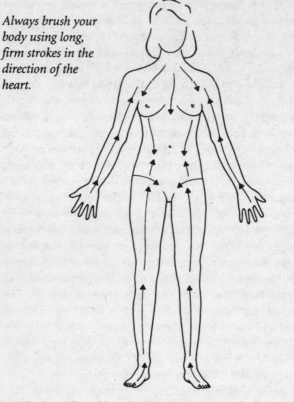

The benefits of dry skin brushing:

* removes dead skin cells and toxins from the body
* stimulates circulation
* is an excellent way of removing cellulite
* stimulates the nerve endings and has a rejuvenating effect on the nervous system, banishing feelings of lethargy or depression
* leaves you feeling totally revitalised!

9

Aromatherapy Detox Massage

As we have seen, herbs play an important part in the process of detoxification. Most of these herbs contain essential oils and each plant has a different oil unique to it, which can be used effectively for all sorts of conditions. All massage is carried out using a basic oil of some description because it makes the hands glide more easily over the skin. But aromatherapy massage is special because this base (or carrier) oil is mixed with a powerful combination of essential oils which can dramatically enhance the effects of the massage. Essential oils have a very small molecular structure which enables them to slip through the skin easily. They are then absorbed into the blood stream and the oil molecules travel through the entire body via an intricate network of blood vessels. This means that they are able to work on the whole body and all its systems until they are eventually excreted through urine, sweat or breath exhalation.

Essential oils have many varied properties. They are all antiseptic, some are antibiotic, others antifungal, antiviral or anti-inflammatory. Some essential oils can stimulate the circulatory system, the lymphatic drainage system, and activate and strengthen the body's own natural immune system. It is these essential oils, of which there are many, which can boost the effects of this detox programme. Essential oils begin their work immediately, first on a patch of skin, then working more deeply in the area and the organs directly beneath the application, and finally throughout the whole body. For a mild effect you can put a few drops of a chosen oil in the bath just before you get in it. You may choose an oil with a relaxing effect before going to bed, and a more invigorating oil at other times. However, the most effective way of using essential oils is to massage them into your skin, applied either to a specific area or your whole body. The massaging itself will stimulate circulation and the lymphatic drainage system, while the essential oil will quickly be absorbed and begin its role in detoxifying your body.

Aromatherapy massage is easy to do and it will certainly make you feel good. There is no need to go to a professional aromatherapist, although this may be more pleasurable, as essential oils are easily available and not complicated to use. However, it must be remembered that just because the oils come from natural herbs and plants, this does not necessarily mean that they are not harmful in large doses. Essential oils should *never* be taken internally and the best way of using them is by adding a few drops of the oil to a carrier oil, such as almond or grapeseed. You can also blend the oils, as many of them have similar effects which work well together. You can either get a friend or loved one to do the massage or do it yourself, although it is hard to reach your own back. The idea of smearing your body with oil may seem unpleasant, but essential oils are unlike other oils as they are neither fatty nor greasy. These plant extracts are volatile, highly flammable and extremely complex. They are wonderfully aromatic and each one has its own individual fragrance. Being volatile means that they evaporate quickly and easily, leaving little or no stain. As for their complexity, essential oils contain hundreds of different chemical components and, as yet, scientists have been unable to reproduce a single one synthetically. The following essential oils are best suited to detoxifying the body:

Basil – this oil produces a similar smell to tarragon and it has been used for centuries to treat jaundice (a condition of the liver) and it aids digestion. Basil also helps to clear mental fatigue, and having a clear, relaxed mind is an important part of any detox programme. This remarkable oil can also improve the tone and appearance of the skin.

Camomile – a wonderfully calming oil which is antibacterial and aids digestion. It has an anti-inflammatory effect, particularly in the digestive system, and is good for diarrhoea and gastritis. Camomile is also very calming on a mental and emotional level which contributes to the body's detoxification.

Cedarwood – this is a very aromatic oil; it is widely used as an incense, and its odour also repels moths and insects. It is a powerful antiseptic and is particularly effective in treating bronchial and urinary infections. Cedarwood has a relaxing effect, and it encourages the elimination of toxins through mucous membranes (these line many cavities including the nasal sinuses, lungs, and pancreatic systems).

Cypress – this oil has a pleasant woody aroma and it is particularly effective in treating water retention as well as boosting circulation. Cyprus also acts as an antiperspirant and deodorant and so could be used instead of these.

Fennel – smells like aniseed and is one of the most antitoxic oils. Fennel is also an excellent carminative and digestive remedy and will relieve the symptoms of nausea, flatulence, indigestion, colic and hiccoughs. It is also a good diuretic and is one of the most valuable oils in the treatment of cellulite.

Juniper – this is another very important oil in the battle against toxins. It has a pungent aroma, but it works well when blended with other oils. It promotes all areas of elimination, and it particularly stimulates digestion and increases the flow of urine.

It is also very good at dealing with cellulite. The cleansing properties of juniper are reputed to work on the mind as well as the body, so it is one of the most thorough detox agents.

Lemon – this oil has a number of important properties, one of which is its ability to stimulate the white blood cells which defend the body against infection. It also neutralises acid in the body which may seem surprising considering its own acid content. Lemon also increases the flow of urine.

Rosemary – the odour of rosemary is similar to that of frankincense. The oil stimulates the central nervous system and the brain and, therefore, helps to clear the mind. It is also an excellent tonic for the heart, liver and gall-bladder.

Tea-tree – this versatile oil does not come from the same plant as the tea which we drink, but from an Australian tree. It has countless different uses, it is antifungal, antibiotic and antiviral. Tea-tree stimulates the immune system and is used therapeutically to help treat disease.

Dosage

Make a blend of some of the essential oils mentioned above by adding a couple of drops of each oil to a bottle of carrier oil such as almond, avocado or grapeseed. (Essential oils should not be added directly to the skin, with one or two exceptions, such as lavender oil.) It is important that you do not add too many drops of any essential oil as this could have an undesirably powerful effect on you.

Adults should use one drop of essential oil to 1ml of carrier oil, ie five drops to every 5ml, ten drops to every 10ml and so on. It is useful to know that 5ml = 1 teaspoon, 10ml = 1 dessertspoon, and 15ml = 1 tablespoon. Do not add more than twenty-five drops of essential oil to 50ml of base oil. Children from the age of seven should use half the adult dosage and increase it gradually until the age of fourteen, when they can use the full adult dosage.

If you want to use essential oils in the bath, add a few drops just before you get in it, as the oils are very volatile and will evaporate quickly. Do not add more than ten drops of essential oil to your bath.

Caution: Do not use essential oils or herbs if you are pregnant without consulting a medical herbalist or trained aromatherapist.

DETOX RECIPE

Add six drops each of the following oils to 50ml of grapeseed, almond or avocado oil: cypress, fennel, juniper and rosemary.

Massage Techniques

The best time to have an aromatherapy massage is after a bath, when the pores of the skin should be clean, open and ready to absorb the essential oils. A relaxed atmosphere with no distracting noises contributes to the benefits of a massage. It is equally important that there are no restrictions on the amount of time you can spend nurturing your body in this way. It is best to have your bath and massage in the evening when you have no other commitments and can go immediately to bed with a relaxed mind and body. Depending on what sort of massage you want, it may be best if you could get a partner to give you the massage, as this allows you to relax your body entirely and let someone else do the work. However, if you want a massage which stimulates the lymphatic drainage system, then this can easily be done alone. Whatever technique you decide on, avoid putting any direct pressure on the breast area or on varicose veins. If you prefer a more professional massage there are many trained aromatherapy masseurs, some of which may even visit your home, for details see Useful Addresses on page 91.

EFFLEURAGE

This technique of massage is designed to have a relaxing effect on both the mind and body. It really needs another person to administer the massage, preferably before bed as the effect is very relaxing. The person being massaged should lie face down, with a cushion placed under the abdomen so that the lower back does not sag. The carrier oil containing your chosen relaxing essential oils should be liberally applied to the feet and calves first and then to the next part of the body which will be massaged. Using basic stroking movements, apply light pressure to each part of the body, moulding your hands to the contours of the tissues. First massage each foot and leg up to the thigh, then each hand and arm up to the shoulder and finish by massaging the whole of the back and neck, starting with the lower back. When concentrating on the back, both hands should travel down the back on either side of the spine, to the middle of the back where they should then follow the line of the ribs to each side of the body. This basic movement should be repeated with a wider gap between both hands each time. When the back of the body has been thoroughly massaged, you can begin work on the front, again starting at the feet and working upwards. Throughout the massage, after the initial general stroking, firmer pressure can be applied, especially to areas which seem to have a lot of built-up tension. This technique of massage is excellent for de-stressing the mind and body and should leave you in a totally relaxed state. Your body is then free to begin its processes of detoxification with no distractions as you sleep.

MASSAGE FOR LYMPHATIC DRAINAGE

This technique has more specific benefits in terms of detoxing your body because it concentrates on stimulating the lymphatic drainage system, and encouraging the removal of toxins through this process. The lymph channels are linked with circulation and are the body's drainage system. Lymph flows through tiny channels which lead to lymph nodes. This is where the lymph is cleansed, and antibodies are released to destroy any foreign invaders which may have entered the lymph. The cleansed lymph is then released into the bloodstream via ducts in the upper body. The more toxic you are and the less exercise you have, the more sluggish your lymphatic drainage system will be which may result in a large build-up of toxins in the lymph.

Contrary to what many writers advise, it is best not to pummel the skin aggressively when attempting to stimulate the lymphatic drainage system, it is far better to use gentle pressure with the hand or just one finger, moving very slowly up the body in the same direction as the lymph itself. If the massage is too vigorous, it will overload the system and may also cause broken blood vessels and bruising. Particular attention should be paid to the lymph glands which are situated in the neck, armpits, backs of the knees and the groin. A mixture of juniper, fennel and cyprus essential oils is a good combination for this type of massage as it will boost circulation and promote the elimination of toxins.

Begin massaging the hands and arms up to your shoulders. Use small, gentle movements, paying particular attention to the lymph glands in your armpits. Then massage each leg up to the groin, using circular movements from the outside of each leg into the groin. The back of each thigh should also be massaged many times, into the groin area. The direction of the massage on the lower back should be outwards from the spine to each side of the body, and on your front you need to massage downwards to your groin. The massage on the upper part of the body (front and back) should be directed towards the nearest armpit. Finally, the neck should be massaged outwards from the centre at the back of the neck, and down the front to the centre of the base of the neck. Study the diagrams below to see the direction of massage more clearly.

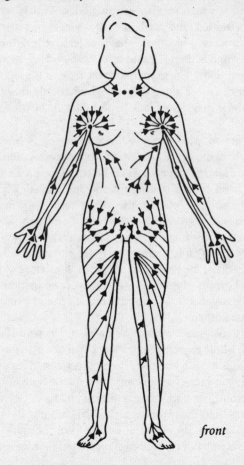

front

The black dots represent the lymph nodes, while the arrows represent the direction in which the lymph flows. Massage along these lines in slow movements to stimulate the lymphatic drainage system.

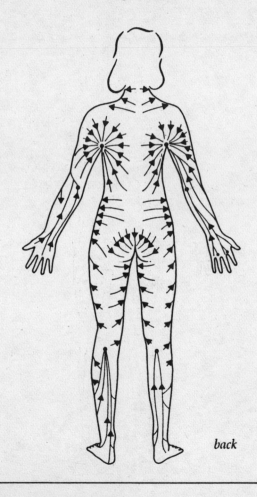

back

—10—

Exercise and Breathing

As we have seen, a large proportion of waste is eliminated from the body via the lungs, and the way in which we all breathe plays an important part in this process. Our breathing also effects the efficiency of the lymphatic drainage system and it is in this respect that breathing and exercise are linked. The circulation of lymph depends greatly on being mechanically pumped by muscle and breathing activity. Anything which you do to improve your breathing and movement through aerobic exercise, stretching or just massage will boost your lymphatic drainage.

Exercise

This is an essential part of the detox programme as it has so many different benefits. We were not designed to lead static lives, where the only movement we make is from the house to the car and from the car to a chair in the office. This daily lack of physical activity will eventually lead to high levels of toxicity in the body and poor health. We need to move our bodies to boost almost every detox process. Without it, our circulation is reduced, our lymphatic drainage is sluggish and our breathing is ineffective. We are also less likely to make full use of the nutrients in our food and our poor lymphatic drainage will lead to a build-up of toxins. The less exercise you have, the more likely you are to feel tired and run down and inclined to find solace in eating chocolate and other comfort foods.

Exercise is also a good mental stimulus as it produces substances called endorphins which are similar to the drug morphine. These help to relieve any pain as well as giving you a natural high. When aerobics became such a popular form of exercise in the early eighties, many women actually became addicted to it and were doing as many as two or more classes a day. Although aerobic exercise stimulates the body in so many different ways, this does not mean that doing it excessively is good for you. Aerobics in particular puts a great deal of pressure on the joints and so it certainly should not be done more than three times a week for more than half an hour each time.

The benefits of regular aerobic exercise are many. It:

* improves the elimination of toxins through the skin by making you sweat

* encourages you to exhale more toxins by changing your breathing patterns

* boosts circulation

* increases heart rate which then carries more fresh nutrients to your cells

* boosts the lymphatic drainage system

* releases endorphins in the brain which give you a sense of well-being

* burns up energy and helps to shed excess body fat

* tones your muscles, giving you a leaner, fitter figure

❋ increases the amount of oxygen which gets to the blood, helping to heal any damage to cells.

There are many different types of exercise that can benefit you which are not quite as demanding as aerobics. Other aerobic exercises such as swimming, cycling, jogging or even walking can be just as good at increasing your heart rate and boosting your circulation. Stretching exercises such as yoga can also have the power to detox your body. To achieve the best detoxing effects, try to exercise continuously for twenty to thirty minutes three times a week on alternate days. This combined with a healthy, balanced diet will give you bags of energy and an enlivened sense of well-being. Try turning mundane everyday activities to your own advantage, by running up stairs and escalators, for example. Put all your energy into walking by taking large strides and using your arms as well. Soon your blood will be pumping through your body at a good rate so that every cell is nourished, leaving your skin glowing with vitality.

WHICH EXERCISE?

If you find aerobics too exhausting and tough on your joints, or swimming in chlorinated pools too sore on your eyes, then there are plenty of other forms of aerobic exercises, one of which is bound to suit your lifestyle and preferences. 'Aerobic' exercise is that which increases your heart rate and the body's ability to deliver oxygen-bearing blood to the muscles and organs. To really benefit from this type of exercise you really need to do it for at least twenty minutes without any break. Sports such as tennis, badminton and squash are not as effective because they involve periods of rest throughout the game. Here are a variety of different exercises to choose from:

Aerobics – it is best to choose low impact aerobics rather than the high impact variety as this is more gentle on your joints, especially if you have not done it before. Almost every health club or sports centre runs aerobic classes and the fact that these organise everything for you is more incentive to go on a regular basis. There are also numerous aerobic workout videos available which you can follow in the comfort of your own home. Before you embark on any aerobic exercise it is vitally important that you do stretching and warming up exercises first as these prepare your muscles for what is in store. If you are suffering from any medical condition which may be affected by exercising, like a sore back, then you should consult your doctor first.

Cycling – this is an excellent form of aerobic exercise which is not tough on your joints, and it will greatly tone your legs. Cycling is also a great form of transport, but not when it is done on busy, main roads where you not only have to stop and start all the time, but you are also breathing in toxic fumes from cars and diesel lorries. Today, of course, you can also cycle in the comfort of your own home on static exercise bikes.

Dancing – exercise does not have to be a repetitive routine of the same short movements, it can be in the form of something which can be enjoyed for itself. Dancing, whether it be disco dancing or ballet, is a much more creative form of aerobic exercise, and it may be something which you already enjoy doing for its own sake. So if you have a busy night life, it is no excuse for not doing any exercise, as the dance floor is the ideal place for some serious blood pumping.

Jogging and running – these two types of exercise really get the blood surging! But they are not suitable for those who have problems with their weight-bearing joints such as knees or ankles. You should avoid running or jogging on concrete pavements or other hard ground as this puts even greater pressure on your joints. Make sure that you wear proper running shoes which provide adequate support and cushioning. If there is a field or park near you then use this, as grass has a certain amount of 'give' which is ideal for this type of aerobic exercise.

Swimming – this is a great exercise for toning your whole body and it does not have the problems which weight-bearing exercises have. When swimming, you are exercising virtually every major muscle in your body but the water keeps you cool. Even those who have weak ankles, knees or back can swim, as your body becomes weightless in water and so removes any pressure on these areas. To get the best out of swimming, you need to swim straight lengths without stopping to rest, for at least twenty minutes. If this is your only exercise, try and do it three times a week, every other day.

Walking – even this everyday activity is aerobic if you put enough energy into it. Either on your way to work or in your lunch hour, you should spend at least ten solid minutes each day walking briskly. As with all other exercises, it is best if you walk in fresh air to ensure that you breathe in large amounts of oxygen and very few toxins. Your body needs oxygen to repair and regenerate its cells, but if you are inhaling plenty of pollution at the same time your body will create free-radicals which cause cell damage.

TONING AND STRETCHING

Stretching exercises will help tone your body and they must be performed before and after each aerobic workout. If you are very stressed or you have not exercised recently, then it is best for you to concentrate initially on just these stretching exercises. If you never take any form of aerobic exercise, then suddenly starting high impact aerobics three times a week will probably reduce you to a severely exhausted state. There are a good many different toning and stretching exercises which you can do instead, all of which can be done at home without exhausting your energy supply or making you hot and sweaty. These exercises will not raise your heart rate significantly, but they are very therapeutic in other respects. Yoga, in particular, is very relaxing and it will help you to control your breathing, enabling you to eliminate more toxins when you exhale. The principles of yoga demand that you perform the exercises slowly, and during each stretch you should take long, deep breaths. As you exhale slowly, you bring your body further into the stretch. Once your body has become accustomed to these gentle, stretching exercises you can combine them with some more active exercises, as it is aerobic exercise which is the key to detoxifying your body.

Breathing

The way in which we breathe is integral to how effectively we eliminate toxins from our bodies. In fact, more toxins are exhaled via the lungs than are passed through urine. Very few of us pay attention to the way in which we breathe and so many of us breathe inefficiently. Instead of making the most of our vast respiratory capacity, many of us walk or sit in a slumped position and are only using our upper chest when we breathe. Breathing properly not only ensures that you are ridding your body of toxins effectively, it also enables you to get an adequate amount of oxygen to the blood. You can follow a simple breathing exercise for five minutes each day, which will boost your energy levels and leave you feeling both relaxed and revived. Lie on the floor on your back somewhere away from distractions, preferably in fresh air. Place a pillow under your knees and rest your hands on your abdomen above the navel. Then take long, deep breaths through your nose to three to four counts, and then exhale slowly through your mouth to the count of four to five. Try and do this simple deep-breathing exercise every day for at least five minutes, perhaps before you go to sleep. If you forget or do not seem to have the time, practise the same deep-breathing technique in the bath or when you are listening to music or in some other relaxed situation.

The Mind–Body Connection

Your mind and body are closely connected, although you may perceive them as two separate entities. Even the tiniest movement your body makes is controlled by your brain, which is why certain diseases of the brain can prevent the patient from moving parts of his/her body. The body easily reveals the state of the mind locked inside it. When a person is feeling tired or stressed, the body often reflects this state through slumped shoulders and a general drooping aspect. This slumped position inhibits our body's digestive function as well as reducing our lung capacity. Similarly, if a person is very happy or excited about something, their body will exude this positive energy in the form of sparkling eyes, a big smile and sprightly movements. Our minds are also the victim of toxins in the form of noise pollution from traffic, car alarms or low flying aeroplanes, and we need to get away from these disturbing distractions for the detox programme to be fully effective. This mind–body link can boost your personal detox if you concentrate your mind on thoughts which help to relax your body, enabling it to perform its detox processes fully. You will find it much easier to eat healthier food, breathe more deeply and exercise if your mind is de-stressed. A short time each day devoted to peaceful meditation will cleanse your mind, while the detox diet, massage and exercise will cleanse your body.

When you have finished this detox programme, your mind and body will be much more in tune with one another. You can easily maintain this level of vitality simply by continuing to eat a healthy, well-balanced diet and exercising. Try to avoid falling back into bad habits and limit your intake of tempting toxic substances such as cigarettes, processed food, caffeine and alcohol. This is just the start of a new, high-energy, healthier way of life.

Glossary

Allergen – a substance which causes an allergic reaction.

Amino acids – nutrients found in foods which are high in protein and which are essential for good health.

Antioxidant – a substance capable of preventing damage to cells by oxidation and free-radicals.

Carcinogenic – a substance known to cause cancer.

Carminative – a substance which relieves flatulence and any gastric discomfort.

Colic – a severe abdominal pain due to an obstruction in the intestine or to constipation.

Diuretic – a substance which increases the flow of urine by promoting the excretion of salts and water via the kidneys.

Essential fatty acids – polyunsaturated fatty acids found in vegetable oils, nuts and seeds which are essential for the good health of all our cells.

Expectorant – a substance which increases bronchial secretion or makes it less viscous. Expectorants are used in cough mixtures.

Flatulence – the elimination of air trapped in the stomach through the mouth, also known as belching or wind.

Free-radicals – highly active and destructive chemical compounds made from oxygen, which cause cell damage.

Laxative – a substance used to cure constipation by increasing bowel movement.

Sensitized – when our bodies become sensitive to a substance or allergen.

Useful Addresses

WHERE TO FIND AROMATHERAPISTS

Send an SAE to the following organisation for a list of locally accredited practitioners:

The Register of Qualified Aromatherapists, 52 Barrock Lane, Aldwick, Bognor Regis, West Sussex PO21 4DD

SUPPLIERS

The following are suppliers of carrier and essential oils. All of them run a mail-order service or, alternatively, would be able to give you a list of local retail outlets:

Aromatherapy Associates, 68 Maltings Place, Bagleys Lane, London SW6 2BY Tel 0171-731 8129/371 9878
Excellent aromatherapy treatments are also available.

Bodytreats, 15 Approach Road, Raynes Park, London SW20 8BA Tel 0181-543 7633

Fragrant Earth, PO Box 182, Taunton, Somerset TA1 3SD Tel 01823-335734

Fleur Aromatherapy, Pembroke Studios, Pembroke Road, Muswell Hill, London N10 2JE Tel 0181-444 7424

Body-brush suppliers

Selected branches of **Boots** and **The Body Shop** or by mail order from:

Green Farm, 225 Putney Bridge Road, London SW15 2PY
Tel 0181-874 1130/5631

Naturopaths

Naturopaths use natural remedies to treat the body as a whole, not just an isolated symptom. Send an SAE for details of your nearest registered naturopath to:

British Register of Naturopathy,
328 Harrogate Road, Moortown, Leeds LS17 6PR

Organic suppliers

The Soil Association,
86 Colston Street, Bath BS1 5BB Tel 0272-290661. Their symbol is a consumer guarantee that food is high quality and genuinely organically grown, ie without the use of pesticides and fungicides. The Soil Association welcomes new members and can also advise on stockists of organically grown produce.

Henry Doubleday Research Association,
Ryton-on-Dunsmore, Coventry CV8 3LG Tel 0203-303517 – This is the largest organisation of organic gardeners in the world and new members are welcome. Products and gardening books are available by mail order.

Index

A

Acidity 57-8
Addresses 91-2
Aerobics 82-4
Alcohol 18, 24, 33
Alfalfa seeds 51, 52
Alkalinity, food 57-8
Almonds 51
Aloe vera 63
Aluminium poisoning 10
Aromatherapy 71-9
Asparagus and mushroom
    risotto 43-4
Aspartame 7-8

B

Bananas, spiced 50
Barley 55
Basil 72-3
Body-mind connection 87-8
Bowel 21-2, 54
Brazil nuts 51
Breathing 19, 86-7
    see also Lungs
Buckwheat 55
Burdock 63

C

Cadmium poisoning 10
Camomile 63, 73
Capsicums 63
Caraway 63-4

Cardamom 64
Cedarwood 73
Chewing 59-60
Chicken with lemon 49
Cinnamon 64
Coriander 64
Cornflour 55
Cycling 83-4
Cypress 73

D

Dancing 84
Dandelion 64
Diabetics 8, 54
Diet 12-3, 24-6
    7-day detox diet 35-8
    21-day detox diet 38-9
    detox diet boosters 51-60
    see also Food combining,
    Meal plans, Recipes

E

Effleurage 76
Epsom salt rub 21
Exercise 81-6

F

Fennel 64, 73
Food combining 58-9
Fruit 8-9
Fruits, detoxifying 36-7

G

Garlic 20, 64-5
Ginger 65
Glossary 89-90
Grains, whole 54-7

H

Hair tonic, anti-dandruff
    15-16
Hazelnuts 51
Heavy-metal toxicity 10
Herbs 62-6
Homeostasis 18-22
Hummus 53-4
Hyssop 65

I

Immune system 17-18
Intestines 21

J

Jogging 83-4
Juniper 65, 73-4

K

Kidneys 20

L

Lemon 65, 74
Liver 19
Lungs 19-20
    see also Breathing
Lymphatic drainage
    and breathing 86-7

and exercise 81-6
massage for 77-9
skin brushing for 67-70
system 22, 67

M

Macaroni and spinach pie 49
Massage 71-2, 75-9
    see also Epsom salt rub
Meal plans 41-50
Mercury poisoning 10
Millet 56
    mash 44
Mind-body connection 87-8
Mushroom and asparagus
    risotto 43-4

N

Nuts 51-2

O

Oats 56
Onion and tofu flan 47

P

Parsley 65, 66
Peanuts 51
Peppermint 66
Peppers, stuffed red 43
Pollutants 9-12, 19
Prawn kebabs 47
Pumpkin seeds 52

Q
Quinoa 55, 56

R
Radiation 11
Recipes 43-4, 46-7, 48-50
Rice 56
Rosemary 66, 74
Running 84
Rye 56

S
Sea vegetables 61-2
Seafood spears 46-7
Seeds 52-3
Sesame seeds 52
Side-effects 32-4
Skin 20-1, 54
    brushing 67-70
    massage 71-2, 75-9
Smoking 19, 24
Spaghetti bolognese 48
Spices 62-6
Spinach and macaroni pie 49
Spirulina 61-2
Stimulants, toxic 26-7
Stretching exercise 83, 85-6
Sunflower seeds 53
Swimming 83, 85

T
Tea-tree 74
Thyme 66
Tofu and onion flan 47

Toning exercise 85-6
Toxic overload quiz 24-9
Toxicity 23-9
    and environment 9-12,
      27-8
    and food 7-9
    at home 14
    in the office 13
    in toiletries 15

W
Walking 83, 85
Walnuts 52
Wheat 54, 57

Y
Yoga 83, 86